CONSIDERING THE
JOURNEY

One Doctor's Perspective

2nd Edition

DR. JEFFREY T. EVANS DHA

CONTENTS

DEDICATION

I am dedicating this book to the memory of my late former spouse and lifelong partner Debbie, who entered into eternal rest shortly before the completion of this book. I spent 43 years with her, 35 married and the rest as partners in life. She would encourage me to pursue my dreams and helped me believe that I could accomplish them. Her encouragement and loving memory will always be in my heart. May she rest eternally in God's arms. This one's for you Deb-Deb.

PREFACE

"Jeffrey, this is Dr. T, now that you have finished your dissertation what do you think will be your next project?" I replied "I want to write a book about the thought process that goes into deciding to pursue a Ph. D or a doctorate degree. I've had several people ask me that question over the past few years and I've had the opportunity to tell it like I see it".

This was how the final moments of the oral defense for my doctorate degree played out after about 15-20 minutes of my presentation. Although I was, at that time, trying to answer the question with the best possible answer I could think of I was voicing the idea for this book. In my preparation for the oral defense, I came across this question several times in researching what type of questions are asked on oral defenses. I honestly didn't think that I had the energy to write a book as my next project after the long seven years it took me to finally finish my doctorate. After writing endless nights during the didactic phase and throughout the process of writing my dissertation I felt that I would never sit in front of a computer and write anything again. But I can honestly say that I started to miss sitting in front of that computer night after night trying to make sense of my thoughts. Seven long years was actually preparing me for the task of writing a book one day, something that I marveled about for many years.

The idea of this book got started as a result of me trying to answer a possible oral defense question from my dissertation. I was advised to figure out what type of project I would like to do after completing my degree. So, I thought that over the past few years I have been asked by friends and colleagues what they should consider when deciding if they should pursue a PhD or doctoral degree. I have advised several that have gone on to begin the journey and a few that decided after they talked to me and saw what I was going through to not start a course.

After finally graduating I became involved with a doctoral support group to help assist those that were going through the journey as a way to give back to the process. I offered my assistance to this group and found out pretty quickly that others in this group had experienced the same thoughts that I had about getting into this program. One of the guest speakers to the group helped inspire me to get started on this book because I felt that this is a message that perspective doctoral candidates needed to hear before making the decision to pursue this degree.

When I came up with the idea for this book there were two other perspective authors that planned to contribute their experiences to give the book more depth. However, due to other commitments they were unable to work with me on this, so I ended up going solo on this project. As a result, the book turned out to be much shorter in length than I originally planned which in my humble opinion makes for a shorter read and more comprehendible for the reader.

The intent of this book is to give the reader a perspective answer to the question of considering the journey, not a thick book breaking down every element and aspect of this question in excruciating detail. A big book might have missed the mark on this. I could have chosen to do more in depth research on this topic as I was taught to do in my doctoral program but I didn't want this to read like an analytical book or quantitative study about the data that describes statistically the breakdown of people that start a program and how many people don't and the many reasons why. That would make for a good study. Actually, there is data out there that shows this breakdown from a statistical standpoint.

I hope that this book helps a perspective student see some of the important aspects of considering the journey and helps them make an informed decision if this is for them or not. If I accomplish that I have met the reason why I put this book in your hand and library. Now sit back and enjoy the journey.

CHAPTER ONE

Introduction

Considering the Journey – One Doctor's Perspective
is a book that reveals the experiences and perspectives
from one doctor's viewpoints of what is referred to as the
"Doctoral Journey". The idea for writing this book came
from many conversations with students, friends, and
perspective doctoral candidates that were considering
pursuing a doctorate or PhD degree but had no idea
of what to expect. What I have found out from these
conversations is that there is a lot that is not commonly
known about the process to attain this level of education.
The majority of people that ask that question had no idea
of what to expect. Many seemed very surprised when I
told them what I had gone through to achieve this degree.
I've also realized that many of the people in the doctoral
or PhD program had no idea of what they were actually
themselves getting into when they enrolled in a program.

For these and many similar reasons are why this
book was written. It is to give a perspective doctoral

candidate an idea of what to expect before signing on the dotted line and committing yourself to "The Doctoral Journey".

This book is written by one doctor that committed himself to this process, continued and finished and has continued to work with doctoral and PhD students in a doctoral support group to help them navigate their way through the doctoral journey.

The doctoral journey is like no other in academia. It is coined the "doctoral journey" in part because it is not like a formal education that you have experienced up to and through the master's level. It generally takes longer than you anticipated and is less regimented than other degrees. Doctoral journeys have been known to add a unique form of stress to a student's life that they were not prepared for or expected when they started the program. The educational counselor conveniently left that out of the conversation when you inquired about the program. The classroom portion of the degree is similar to previous degree work with reading assignments, discussion and projects on a timeline that are graded and returned. But the dissertation side can be long and unregimented and due to circumstances beyond your control can take longer than you anticipated. A common phrase that is used to describe this portion of the degree is commonly referred to as the "dissertation blues".

Despite all the headaches that come up during this process, the achievement of being called "Doctor" at the end of the journey is a rewarding and well worth the work accomplishment in one's life.

The intent of this book is not to deter someone from pursuing their dreams of accomplishing a doctoral or PhD degree by talking negatively about the rigors of achieving this level of education, but to rather prepare them mentally for what to expect before they make the commitment to beginning the journey. The journey's end is not always guaranteed to be successful, nor is it always the journey that you anticipated from the beginning. However, the better prepared you are to make the journey the better your chances are for succeeding in the journey.

With that thought in mind, the degree completion rate for doctoral degrees is somewhat different than it is for lesser level degrees. Several studies have been done over the past decade in the United States which puts the completion rate somewhere between 50 and 60 percent. There are several factors that these studies have determined to be the reasons why certain degree programs were not completed. The intention here is not to examine these studies in depth but to point out that this is a factor to consider when deciding if this is a degree that you want to pursue. When examining the available literature about completion rates there seemed to be more articles about the doctoral and PhD level than there was for undergrad and master's degrees. I drew the assumption for this to be because the program is different in many ways from the traditional master's and undergrad degree programs. I also bring this up because I have encountered several people in doctoral programs that are "All But Dissertation" (ABD) and have not finished and seem to be stuck in a void. Some schools have the candidate work on the dissertation within the curriculum while some save the dissertation work for the end of the program. The dissertation is a long tedious process that takes time and has been known to be the main reason why many don't finish these programs.

Since the dissertation phase is at least one half of the program, I am focusing most of this book on that experience. It is a unique experience and one that should be known to the perspective doctoral candidate before the journey begins. The class study and dissertation phase are two totally different phases of the program. The more you know ahead of time the better prepared you will be when the time comes to start working on it. During the course work you will likely cover courses that deal with the components of the dissertation and will become very familiar with them over time. The program I went through did just that. Some of my earlier courses were about research and how to conduct it. The residencies reinforced that by working out problems and actually working on parts that will later be used on your dissertation.

These were invaluable classes because your best bet is to have a thorough understanding of the components before you begin and not try to play catch up as you go along. Trying to learn something and do it at the same time will only slow down your progress through the program.

With all of this in consideration it is almost pertinent that a perspective doctoral candidate have some insight into this process before beginning this program.

CHAPTER TWO

Why My Journey Began

The journey begins with an idea or a dream. A mentor or authority figure in your life has achieved this level of education and you begin to wonder how they did it. What does it take to accomplish a degree at this level? Sometimes the idea or dream begins with the expectations of parents and family members. They see some potential in you, and they express their thoughts to get you thinking about it. Your occupational field can sometimes require that you attain this level of education in order to enter into the level that you have chosen to work at, or you just feel it is necessary to go this far with your education because you want to. There are many reasons why someone pursues this level of education, and the reason is as unique and individual as the person that applies to a program.

Whatever the motivation is that gets you interested in pursuing this degree it must be strong enough to make the journey. It has to sustain your motivation to continue to work against what seems like all odds and against any and all adversity that obstructs your path. The journey is not easy and obstructions are intended to make you work hard and to persevere through what might seem like endless and meaningless hurdles. However meaningless it may seem there is a rhythm to the madness. There is a reason why it is designed this way. I'm not going to tell you about the reasons for this, however this is where I will suggest that if you want to find out then you must complete a doctoral or Ph. D program. This is an exclusive club and the only way into it is to complete the journey. I leave you there for some motivation.

My journey started way back in the first grade. My sister (4 years older) was very good in school whereas I was just getting started but was being compared to her by my mother. My first report card was mostly B's and my mother asked me why was there all B's and not A's. She assumed that I was playing in school and not doing my work and scolded me for it. She was used to seeing all A's on my sister's report cards and assumed that mind would look the same. She hadn't experienced a B student in her family yet and really wasn't prepared to see one at the time. That incident stayed with me well into my adult years and is probably the main motivator as to why I considered the journey. The motivation for the journey started from the day when I was six years old in the first grade and continued until I finally started the doctoral journey when I was 52 years old, some 46 years later. Along the way I achieved an associate degree in Environmental Health, a bachelor's degree in Business Management and a master's degree in Health Services Management. These three degrees spanned over some 16 years. I honestly didn't have a rock-solid plan when setting my sights on these degrees other that the associates degree from a school where I was studying for my occupational field at the time. The bachelor's and master's degrees were requirements for the career path I had chosen while in the Navy. After attaining my master's degree in 1994 I honestly thought that was as far as I was planning to go educationally for the rest of my life. I was satisfied at that level and felt that there was no way that I would go back to school again. What I didn't know at the time was that the fire to keep going was still burning inside me.

Well the motivation wasn't gone yet. After 1994 I began coaching little league football and really loved it. I thought that this was my calling and that I had found something to satisfy my thirst to be doing something. I did this for several years before deploying to Iraq with the Marine Corps. For two summers I was unable to coach because of work commitments. In total I coached for 12 years before the bug for going back to school bit me again. A good friend kept talking to me about going back to school to pursue a doctorate or PhD. I disregarded this for several reasons. First and foremost, I said that I would never go back to school again. Secondly, I didn't want to devote the time after work to studying again and lastly, I wanted to keep on coaching. During the off season from football one day, I received an email from the University of Phoenix about going back to school and for some reason didn't delete it, leaving it in my inbox. One of my sons came to me to talk about motivation and life in general. We took a trip about 60 miles away to a mall and had lunch and just generally talked about life and how to navigate it. When I got home that night at around 12:00 midnight I got on my computer and filled in the information on the University of Phoenix email and sent it in. The conversation ended up motivating me more than it did my son. Two days later the University of Phoenix contacted me and the journey began. I just jumped into it really not knowing what I was getting myself into. Financially, I still had some of the G.I. Bill available and was hoping that it would cover it. As far as what to expect from the course I had no idea. I wasn't pursuing a doctoral degree for my occupation or needing it for a job requirement, I was just doing it for myself to see if I could do it and subconsciously to show my mother (who was 83 years old at the time) that I can work hard in school and get good grades. That stayed with me for a long time and my goal was to finish my doctorate degree before my mother left God's green earth for greater pastures. I accomplished that goal when she was 90 years old, some seven years after I began.

So, you can see from this short story that my motivation was probably different from yours and most likely different from most. Whatever it is that motivates you it must be able to sustain you while on the journey. You must have something that keeps you going when your brain is telling you to give up. We all have a different perspective of what we perceive a doctoral program to be like.

Why?

The first question that should come to mind should be, why do I want to do this? Why do I want to devote so much time and effort to getting a doctorate or PhD? The reasons are numerous and as personal as the person you are asking. The number of answers to this question would probably fill up this book if I asked enough people. Could the reasoning process not have all the information needed to process a desire like this idea? There's a good chance that this is a factor that has been considered unless you are the type that does their own in-depth research on this before you decide to get into it.

I personally didn't do much research and I would be willing to bet that most that get into these programs haven't done the research as well. I've come to this conclusion based on my experiences and the conversations that I've had with doctoral candidates that were in my residencies and the cohort that I am a part of.

Another question you might ask yourself is, what is the importance or significance of having a doctoral degree or PhD? What's the difference in my life if I have one or not? Will it change my status on the job, in academia, in my community or just within myself? Is it something that I am willing to sacrifice my time and money to achieve if it isn't going to change much other than increase my student loan? Is it going to improve my status at work and put me in line for a considerable promotion? Will my employer take notice and improve my position at work and give me bigger oversight or more responsibility?

Will a doctoral or PhD open doors to opportunity for me that wouldn't necessarily be opened without it? Are these doors something that I can and want to live with? Some people gain more responsibility at work and then later realize that they were not cut out for something this after the fact.

A doctorate degree or PhD can change your life probably more than a lesser degree can. A colleague once told me, while I was just starting out in the program, that if someone asks you a question as a doctor that they feel that whatever you say is correct. I understand the gest of this statement to mean that since you have "doctor" in front of your name that you are likely to have an educated answer to their question and they will abide by what you tell them. With this title comes an expectation that others will have of you. Some of us aren't used to that but might want to become with this concept just in case this happens to you.

People have the picture in their mind that you have been through an extensive educational program to become a doctor and that you have to be smarter than the average to even get into the program. For me personally, I thought the same thing for a long time. Now having gone through the program I see it differently than I did before. There is an acceptance criterion that you have to go through to get into a program, but I don't think they are just looking for the cream of the crop smart people. I think they are looking at your experience and how well you have been able to be successful in what you do. My program had to have a few letters of reference from people in your field along with the package for acceptance. They also considered my past transcripts as do all colleges before they will accept you. I had this idea in my head that my previous grades would not be high enough to get me accepted. My grades were good but not a 4.0 GPA.

There are several other criteria that schools look at in order to consider you for their program. That was an eye opener for me because I've always thought that there was no way that I would get into a doctoral or PhD program because of my grades not being high enough. That is just something that I have always heard and never gave it much thought until I decided to try to get into a program.

Truth be known I had no idea what I was getting myself into, neither did I have any idea about the application process until I received a call from the university. Applying to a program for me was a complete shot in the dark. I wanted to get accepted but wasn't putting all my money in that one pot. If I got in, great, but if I didn't it wouldn't have been a big disappointment for me since I really didn't think I would. Taking the stress from me to get in probably was a blessing in disguise since there was no pressure riding on the decision. There was no support unit that was pushing me to do it or not. Unlike the young 18-year-old coming out of high school trying to get into a specific college I didn't have to worry about all of that.

After that first phone call from the school and the representative helped build my confidence that this was something that I could do I was off to the races. The application process wasn't as hard or scary as I thought it would be and with a little confidence from the beginning, I came to expect that I would be accepted. After a few short weeks all the paperwork was in, and I was cleared for my first class.

The first class was a short three-week class with a million assignments designed to give you a taste of time management and how much time you will be spending on class and home work. Some people refer to this class as "boot camp" as it was getting you ready for the rigorous path ahead. I went through an online program that, in my opinion, you have to be more disciplined for. It was my first online schooling experience, and I am so glad now that I chose to challenge this route. For me, it was easy for me to stay on track on my own rather than having an instructor telling me what to do in a classroom. Many of my colleagues at the residencies that I attended felt the same since many were working students and had jobs and families to tend to. The online class gave me the flexibility to snap in when I was ready to and to not be in a classroom at a specific time on a given day.

After the boot camp phase, the classes began to get increasingly more demanding in terms of time requirements and assignments. The boot camp class was a teaser compared to the classes that followed. After about four to five courses the classes that support writing the dissertation started. This prepared you for the first residency where we would discuss the framework of whichever method you decided to use, qualitative or quantitative. In the big picture this was a good way to approach writing a dissertation. In this curriculum you were already working on your dissertation before classes ended.

In the decision process of whether to pursue a doctorate or PhD degree you have to weigh the pressure of writing the dissertation. Little might be known by the perspective candidate in the very beginning other than what you might have heard from friends or colleagues. The dissertation process is a challenge all by itself.

The class work is also a challenge, but it is one that you have already experienced in your previous degree work. The dissertation, depending on the school and its requirements, is something that should be closely examined before signing on the dotted line.

I was taken completely by surprise with the dissertation process because I failed to do my research about the process before I applied. I had heard the horror stories of people talking about their experiences but had never questioned them or bothered to investigate it before I started.

There is something to be said about this approach that doesn't make it totally wrong on my part. I once had a boxing coach ask me if I wanted to become a boxer when I was in the Navy. My reply to him was that I didn't know anything about boxing and that I had never boxed before. He told me that that was the perfect type of person he was looking for because he preferred to teach someone who didn't know anything as opposed to teaching someone who knew a little and thought they knew a lot. He said that he would have to break their bad habits and teach them all new ones in order to become a good boxer.

For me, challenging this program from that perspective was probably a plus in my favor because I hadn't formed an opinion based on other people's thoughts. I didn't hear any negative thoughts that helped form my thoughts. If I had gotten a dose of negativity from others regarding this program I might have gone into it with the wrong mindset. The program is hard enough and really doesn't need anything else to be negative or hard to do.

This is somewhat contradictive for the reason why I wrote this book, but I do believe that the more you know from an unbiased viewpoint the better you will be prepared to deal with the rigors of this program. It probably would have not hurt me to do a little research before I got myself knee deep in the program before I realized what I got myself into. At the least I think I would have been a little more prepared for what to expect as I got deeper and deeper into the program.

I also think that success in a program has something to do with the type of person you are. What I mean is that you have to be able to adapt to the way things happen in a program. There will be numerous setbacks that can play havoc on your timetable to finish the course. You have to learn early on how you will choose to deal with these setbacks. A perfectionist may have big problems because they expect everything to be perfect or as they planned it. These setbacks arise when an instructor or committee member doesn't see things the way you do and their expectation needs to be met not yours.

An example of that happened to me is when I had to retake a class because I had to withdraw due to medical reasons. When I retook the class the first assignment was the same as it was in the previous class that I had withdrawn from. So, I changed the dates and submitted the paper for the subsequent class. The instructor blasted me for what he called dovetail plagiarism. I had never heard of dovetail plagiarism before and was caught completely off guard when the instructor contacted me and threatened to charge me with an academic penalty for it.

Retaking a class was already a setback that I didn't expect but to add to it an academic charge for resubmitting my own paper was a lot for me to swallow. I was totally innocent about the plagiarism and was able to explain myself out of that one, but it put a bad taste in my mouth. After this happened I stuck to my own teaching and was committed to turning a negative thing positive and didn't complain about it but rather turned this energy into pushing harder and did well in this class as a result of this incident.

Another hurdle that comes in almost every doctoral candidate's journey is not staying on course to finish when you decided you wanted to. "You" being the key word here. You have a plan, but your plan must fit into everyone else's plans that are a part of your committee or part of the program. Here is where problems that you can't fix, or answer come up and you just must deal with them. Choose to be upset or just keep plugging away are the choices you get so choose wisely. These programs have milestones that you have to meet in order to push through the program and stay on course. Some of the setbacks that I am referring to happen around these milestones.

For me, I got hung up on one that probably should have never happened, but it did and had to deal with it. If I was determined to finish at a particular time, then this setback would have been disastrous for me and really added a lot of stress to my life. I didn't take it to heart, but I did notify my chair and the school to get it taken care of. It honestly set me back about a year in my plans to finish at a specific time.

Other setbacks come from everyday life and the things that can happen to you over the course of your time in the program. Some of these things can be moving to a new location due to a work change or requirement, the birth of a child, the death of a family member, a divorce or a number of things that take up your time and effort and make it too hard for you to continue on the same pace you are on. You have to be ready for these and plan ahead and how to stay on course as they come up.

For me, I had a personal family issue and a death in the family that took a lot out of me but didn't knock me off course. During one of my residencies, we talked about this in class, and I was amazed at how much these things affected people. When I thought that it was few and far between, I found out that it affected at least one out of five in the classroom and cohort that was going through at the time. So, when you think it's only happening to you, think again. This is much more common than you think it is.

The main thing you need to know about setbacks is that when they happen you have to find a way to get through them and get back to work. It's hard to do that sometimes but a must that needs to be done. Bouncing back from a setback relies a lot on your motivation to get through the program. What does it take to get you back in the game and on the journey again when you have to stop for a while. I talked earlier about motivation and how to use it to keep you going. Well, this is an instance where that motivation is needed to keep you going.

I've had colleagues in the program that have been faced with big life changing setbacks that just needed some outside motivation to get them back in the game. I've also seen those that just couldn't find a way to keep going and dropped from the program. Ultimately, realizing that this can happen to you and how you deal with it can be a major game changer on the journey.

CHAPTER THREE

Considerations

Before you embark on a trip, or in this case a journey, you have to prepare for the time it takes to get there, the time you will spend there, and the plan to get back. In this case, you have to plan for the time it takes to get there. What you do when you get there isn't included necessarily at this time in the plan. In preparing for the journey you will have your hands full with each phase that you wouldn't have room for any other phase as you progress through the process.

To help you with your planning I have picked out a few areas that I would strongly recommend that you take some time to examine and get a good sense of where you are at with them. These are some of the major areas that play an important part in how well you navigate through the journey. I will discuss how I dealt with each area and hope that I cover enough ground for you so that you get the main idea and can formulate how you can deal with each area.

Some of these considerations I gathered from conversations with doctoral candidates and doctors about how they dealt with similar situations. For each person the way you deal with the situation is totally yours and no one else's. Everyone has their own way of dealing with their issues and this is no different.

The big difference with this I believe is that there are not a lot of people going through a doctoral or PhD program that you can talk to when things come up. People who choose to pursue this degree are not the norm, they are the more ambitious and determined people because of the time and effort it takes to achieve this goal.

Finances

Finances for school can come in many different ways, i.e. student loans, out-of-pocket, financial plans from specific schools or the good old-fashioned parents pay for your education way. Whatever the method of payment, a doctorate or PhD is an expensive degree and will cost someone lots of money.

When it came to finances, I was very fortunate. For me, finances weren't a big problem because I had substantial financial support from the Viet Nam Era G.I. Bill left over from my active-duty days. As a retired veteran I qualified for financial aid that essentially paid for 95% of my degree. Some schools, like University of Phoenix, require the student to attend several residencies at the home campus. The University of Phoenix required three with the strong possibility of a fourth. I attended four residencies. The residency for me was the cost of a plane ride, a hotel room, and the cost of the course. The residencies lasted between 3 to 8 days depending on which one it was. The cost of lodging and flights were not covered under the G.I. Bill but were out of the pocket costs. So, cost of financial concerns must be taken into consideration beyond the cost of classes and must be within your proposed budget for school. Costs can easily escalate beyond expectations depending on how many "extra" classes you might have to take. An example of an "extra" class would be if you failed to submit your dissertation for review in the allowed or required time period and need to take an additional class so that you would be in a class to meet the submission requirements. Life happens and sometimes these "extra" classes are required and not initially accounted for. In my case, I had to take two additional classes, one a class and the other a residency, due to needing to update the version of program that I was in and to meet a submission requirement. These two additional courses cost me about $5,000 dollars, which included the air fare to and from Phoenix and the hotel costs for three days.

Budgeting for what you expect costs to be and the unforeseen must be accounted for. Once you are knee deep in the dissertation process you may need to put out additional costs to have your proposal edited by an editor that charges and you might decide to have your data analyzed by an outside source to ensure that it is done right. These costs can begin to add up and are not apparent from the beginning.

Another approach to financing a post graduate degree is to take a student loan out to cover the cost. Student loans are low interest, long term loans that allow a student to pay them off over a longer than usually period of time. I personally don't have any experience using a student loan but have been associated with several friends and colleagues that have used them over the years.

One friend of mine had a student loan that seemed to hang over their head for many years. I would say for about 6-7 years my friend would constantly mention that that was their goal to pay off their student loan. I don't know what the monthly payment was or what the amount of the loan was for, but I do know that it was for a substantial time period. This particular friend used their student loan for a master's degree and several other classes they took towards a certification.

Another one of my friends used a student loan towards a doctoral degree and shared their experience with me. My best guess is that they used the loan to pay for the entire degree because of the way they talked about it when they first started out and how the amount owed grew over time. With no other financial support, the loan paid for the entire degree. My friend told me that when the loan grew to over $100K they began to get a little disillusioned because the total owed was growing and they weren't getting satisfaction from the work they were putting into it. They were in the dissertation process and all of the setbacks on "the journey" were not worth the amount of money that as going out and continuing to grow. The frustration was growing and it began to seem that it wasn't worth the hassle to continue. Another factor was that their significant other put a little pressure on the situation because of all the money that was going out into the loan was creating a long-term debt that they were beginning to wonder if it would ever get paid off. Rightfully so the significant other didn't want to throw money away that they wouldn't see any return on investment on.

I have had several motivational conversations with this friend over the past few years to keep them motivated to continue and finish the journey. I believe that owing that large amount of money with nothing to show for if they dropped out kept my friend motivated to continue. They haven't finished yet but have continued to push on through the hard times to keep the motivation to finish.

My takeaway from this is that if you have to take out a student loan be aware of the long time debt it puts on you and how you can use it for motivation when times get tough. Having any kind of (negative) debt isn't necessarily a good thing but can be used as a motivator when you need something to keep you going. I can't imagine what it must feel like when you have a large long time loan debt hanging over your head and have decided to drop out of the program. That to me would be like throwing money out of a window. Interestingly, with the incompletion rate for this level of education at about 50% that's a lot of money that is being paid out and not getting a return of their investment.

Another financial approach would be to pay for it yourself through periodical payments over a period of time. This would probably be the most sensible way if you can afford it. This would give you control over your finances and leave you little debt to worry about at the completion of the degree if you could stay on track and pay for it in full as you go through the curriculum. That would likely be a very costly venture doing it this way but gives you a good sense of mind financially as you are going through the program. With courses ranging from anywhere between $2K and 3K a class this could get pretty costly to pay for out of pocket.

I have a colleague that is paying for their degree this way and concurs with my observation above. I can honestly say that I have never heard that person complain about paying for the program. That tells me that they must have a pretty good system down for making payments and being sure that they stay on track with their classes.

I would add that if that is the way you choose to pay for your degree that you be very conscientious about paying your bills and don't fall behind. Obviously, colleges are business institutions and will not tolerate late payments while you are on the journey. Again, this is a very good motivator in case you start to fall behind your schedule and need something to pick you up.

I also learned from my friend that paying for the program this way also took some of the stress of finishing off of her shoulders because she literally paid as she went. She told me early on that she was in no hurry to finish and that this slowed her down to the pace that she was comfortable with. She could take a planned break between classes to catch up on things in her life that she was neglecting while in class. This gave her a clear picture of where she was going and how she planned to get there.

She hasn't finished yet but is solidly on her way. She told me her goal was to finish with little or no debt on the books for her degree and to not stress out along the way. These sound like some pretty good goals if paying for your degree out of pocket is the way you plan to finance it. The big thing here is that you have to be patient and able to stay motivated if you choose to take a break or two from classes along the way.

Time Management

Another area under consideration to look at is time management. When I started my journey, the first class I took was about time management, how to effectively manage the time you have to get everything done that you have to get done. Adding night courses to your already busy work/family life is a challenge that must be negotiated. Most people that have a master's degree have pretty much figured out the study time issue with their significant other or living environment. So, for the course work part of the degree that has already been figured out. The writing of the dissertation is the added part that depending on the school could be started during regular courses or as some schools still do it, after the course work is done. My advice here is to go to a school that believes in starting the dissertation while you are still taking courses and not put it off until all course work is completed.

The dissertation process is a totally different entity all to itself. I never wrote a thesis in my master's degree, but I've talked to people that have that have written a dissertation or were in the process of writing it and they told me hands down that the dissertation process is a lot more challenging. Writing my dissertation took me ten times more time to work on than any class I took.

When I was planning to go back to school for my doctorate, I was told to expect to need about 20 hours a week devoted to studying on top of my normal work week. That equated to about 3.5 hours a day, 7 days a week added for reading assignments, doing homework and posting online. For me that turned out to be about 30+ hours a week devoted to my studies. So you can see from my experiences that time does play an important factor into what you can get done in the time you have.

I'd put the commitment to time high on the list of considerations when deciding on whether to make the journey or not because this is a life-changing event and will undoubtedly change the way you live your life for a few years. My social life and personal life changed drastically because I devoted all of my time to my studies. I had very little time for extracurricular activities, including my passion for watching pro football games on Sundays, during my first 4 years in the program. As I look back on it now, I'm not sure how I did it. It was a complete change of my mindset that allowed me to make it through those years while I was on the journey.

The time commitments for writing my dissertation were almost double what I had planned for during my class work. The dissertation is very time consuming, and the system will not allow you to cut any corners when writing it. The requirements are very specific, and anything less will not make it through the process. Therefore, my point here is that after your class work is done be prepared to spend even more time writing your dissertation. This is the part of the journey where motivation is needed at times to keep you going.

While you are writing your dissertation you will find out that you don't even control the time after you submit it for corrections because you are submitting it to a committee that have personal lives as well. You will be subjected to their time management skills in correcting and returning your paper and will be given timelines to get the corrections done and returned for review. You must learn to be flexible during this time in order to not lose your mind over what you cannot control. This can get nerve racking if you allow it to so be careful and pace yourself and use expectation management along with time management to be successful during this time. I almost let it drive me crazy during this time in my program until I finally figured this out.

Family/Personal Life

The next consideration to examine would be your family life and where you are at with that. The time commitment can take you away from your normal routine of family time because of the projects and deadlines that you will be required to meet. Going through your master's degree gave you a good perspective of what to expect for the course work of a doctorate degree but the dissertation phase is totally different. The dissertation phase is self-paced and directed. The time constraints come in when there are deadlines to meet for submissions or imposed by your committee chair to meet certain milestones. Much of the dissertation phase is consumed with doing research, writing, collecting and analyzing data. Each of these can take a great amount of time and effort to accomplish.

Family time and involvement can be a factor if that is something that is important to you. It would be a good idea to sit down and have frank and honest conversations with family members with whom would be affected by your absence if you decided to go back to school. Young children might not understand why their parent is not spending much time with them and a significant other might have a hard time grasping this idea as well. So, it is pertinent that everyone involved knows up front what to expect before you start on this endeavor. Honest feedback is encouraged because a certain amount of guilt of not spending time could be an Achilles heel once you get started. Once the green light is on with all involved then my recommendation would be to discuss how family time will be spent so that everyone involved knows where they stand and what to expect while you are in school. Also, after you discuss it make sure that you make do with what you planned so that no one feels left out once you start school. Talking about your plan and carrying out the plan could be two different things so make sure that you keep your word.

Personal life for someone that is single or not married is of major concern as well. Depending on how you like to spend your free time or after work time this program can be very time consuming and cut down on the amount of time you have to yourself. The number of hours devoted to studying is the same for the single person as it is for the married person. Therefore, the time commitment is relatively the same. However, the amount of time that you have for personal activities becomes very limited and one that you must get used to once you are in the program. I lived by myself for the entire program, and I had almost no time for personal activities much less a life outside of my studies. I'm an avid football fan and I can say that I didn't watch an entire football game for the first three years while in the program. It would be smart to prepare your mindset for this before you get into the program to give yourself time to make the adjustment once you start.

Since finishing my degree I've had friends and co-workers come to me for advice about going into a program. One of the first things that I ask them is about their family life and how many people are in their family. Based on their answer I try to give them an honest assessment and opinion of what to expect if they make the decision to pursue the program. I have a co-worker that is a very driven and ambitious person who came to me for advice. She is a single mother with three children. The youngest I believe she said was about 4 or 5 years old. The other two are 8 and 11 years old. Based on this I told her what I could imagine would be her biggest challenge, spending quality time with her kids. At that age I know from having a family myself that you as an adult must devote a lot of time to a child's upbringing. They require a lot of your time. Going through a doctoral program requires a lot of your time as well. So, you would have competing priorities that could circumvent each other.

My advice to her was reconsider going back to school at this time and to put off this goal when her kids got older. She didn't quite understand why I advised her in this manner because she had always been an "A" student and did very well in the didactic studies that she has experienced. I tried to explain that a doctoral or PhD was a different type of program and that she would experience a much different curriculum than she has been used to. Up to the dissertation for her would be similar to what she was used to in master's degree, but the dissertation phase would be much different than what she was used to and could present a problem.

We talked extensively about it and came to the conclusion that she could go ahead and challenge it but I felt and advised her that it would probably take her a longer time to complete the program than if she didn't have the family to take care of. I say this because there will inevitably be times where she will have to make the decision to either work on getting some work on her dissertation done or take the time to spend it with family. In my opinion, I could see this happening more than not which would slow down her progress in the program.

So, this brings me to timing and when is the best time to enter a program. Many would say that there really is no best time to make the move, but I respectfully would disagree with them because I feel that you have to plan for your success and not just stumble into it.

Timing can be as simple as planning the program when you think that you would have the least distractions. Now don't get me wrong, family time is not a distraction. What I mean is that planning when you would have the least number of things on your plate to do is what I am talking about. Raising a family is very important and raising it to the best of your ability is a high priority. Working a full-time job while going to school is a big demand on your time and adding in the raising of a family is an even bigger demand. Having too much on your plate can set you up for failure if you make the wrong move and the wrong time.

So, my best advice with this is to be honest with yourself about how well you think you can balance a full schedule and then decide how you would negotiate this if you decide to pursue the program. If you have a young family and don't really need the degree of career development or promotion then I would strongly advise that you wait until your family is older and you have more time to work on the degree. If having a doctorate or PhD is not needed in your immediate future, then I would venture to say that there really is no hurry to get it. I was 59 years old when I walked across the stage and I wasn't the oldest person in the residencies that I attended. Going back to why you want or need the degree should lend some indicators about when to pursue the degree. Putting "Dr" in front of your name doesn't magically make a couple hundred thousand dollars appear in your paycheck. It helps in your career but is not the magic formula for making it at a specific time in your career. In some cases that isn't always true but for the average person in the program it probably is closer to the truth. So, I say that because as the saying goes, "haste makes waste" and you sure don't want to make waste in a program that costs what a doctoral or PhD costs.

Family is just one of the variables to consider in this decision, but I would put it close to the top because you just can't get family time back. But you can use good timing and adjust your game plan and accomplish a doctoral or PhD later in life. The timing of your pursuit for this degree is totally up to you as to when you plan to begin the journey. Your reason for doing this should have some bearing as to when you plan to get it done (i.e., career, personal reasons, self-betterment). Therefore, let this reason dictate what your plan will be to begin.

Career

Another consideration would be your career. People enter this journey for many reasons, one of which might be your career. A doctoral degree might be the ticket to a higher level of income or job requirement that is needed to continue in your chosen field of work. If this is the case I'd say that this is very solid and good motivation to pursue this degree. Wanting to climb the proverbial corporate ladder or accomplish a specific level in your work is a noteworthy reason to enter this type of program.

For me that wasn't the case and for many others that attended residencies with me not many were trying to meet career requirements. I found it interesting that so many were doing it for themselves and for the challenge. There was a doctoral candidate in one of my residencies that was 65 years old and retired from two careers. His motivation was self-imposed and was just a personal goal he had made for himself many years before retiring. Career and work got in his way and he just never got started early on.

A career goal is a very good reason to start the journey and one that should keep someone motivated throughout when it seems impossible to continue. There will be days when continuing seems improbable and you begin to dig for reasons to continue. This is when a very good reason to finish should be relied upon to bridge that gap to keep going.

One thing to keep in mind here is that career goals could put some pressure on you to finish in a specific time period. This is one of my pet peeves, pressure. Putting a finish deadline on yourself can put you under a certain amount of pressure to finish. Once you begin your dissertation there are timelines that have to be met and sometimes you have no control over meeting them. For instance, turning your paper over to your chair/committee for review doesn't always mean that you will get it back when you want to. They have lives and commitments and reading and correcting your dissertation might not be on the priority list for several days or weeks for them. You have absolutely no control over this.

During my journey one phase took over a year to complete and it was totally out of my control. If I had a self-imposed due date, it would have driven me crazy because it wouldn't have been met on time.

So, I say all of this to say that be careful on the deadlines that you put on yourself and realize that at some point you will not be able to control the outcome. A career goal is good but can impose deadlines on you that only turn up the pressure and make things worst that they really are. Be realistic and accept things the way they are and you will succeed in all that you have planned for this journey in a timely manner.

Another thing about career goals is that your career could be riding on you finishing at a certain waypoint and there is a must that you make that waypoint or else you lose out. That can be a risky venture if you are betting on someone else's time to meet your goals. Give yourself a cushion for the unexpected just in case you run into some hurdles along the way which will most likely happen. I can't think of one person that didn't experience some hurdles that slowed them down along the way to finishing.

Career goals can be pressure and believe me you don't need anymore pressure on you once you get into the dissertation phase. So, make the career goals doable, understand the hurdles and keep pressing on once you get into the program.

Ambition

Ambition can play an important part of why someone wants to make the journey. Ambitious people by nature have a desire to challenge and accomplish a goal, regardless of how lofty it might seem or be. Ambition might be the only reason why someone takes on this challenge.

For me, I had an ambition to become a doctor someday. I had no idea what I was going to do to get there and didn't think I was smart enough to even challenge the entrance tests to go to medical school. So, I wasn't sure what type of doctor I was going to become. When I was in my senior year of high school I would tell my friends that I wanted to get a doctorate in psychology one day. It was really just talk back then but now that I think about it, it was probably an ambitious way of saying that it really was my goal one day to do so. When I was about two thirds through my Navy career, I attended Johns Hopkins University for a 3-week course in my career field. During the course, I became acquainted with one of my fellow students and we talked about becoming doctors in our chosen profession one day. I believed again that it was in my ambitious DNA but had no idea how I would get there. As I got older the thought of going back to school again started to fade with coaching football and with retirement from the military coming soon. But, that ambitious side of me didn't stop and I was finally shown the way to the journey and started it was I was 52 years old and finished it at 59 years old. So, this just goes to show that being ambitious could over-rule age and doubts and put you on the road to making the journey one day.

Being ambitious is a feeling that harbors deep down inside someone and is defined by that individual's desire to succeed at something that is a challenge to them. For me that ambitious feeling kept burning inside me and finally came to fruition as I got older. Although it was just talk among friends at an early age I believe that deep down inside me there was a fire burning that could only be extinguished by pursuing my dream and one day completing a doctoral program. I never thought that I would achieve this level of education but the ambition I harbored kept that feeling alive.

Over the years I have been witness to several of my friends achieving a PhD and can remember them talking about how long it took them and how much they had to put into it. I honestly never thought that I would be among them one day because I couldn't see myself going through all that they did. Again, I didn't think that I was smart enough to even challenge a program's admission process and didn't think or have the confidence in myself to even envision it.

My ambition somehow kept me going to pursue it and finally paid off when I finally challenged the admissions process. As I got confirmation that I was getting accepted into the program my enthusiasm and confidence started to grow. Something that I have only dreamed of was finally becoming a reality. I never thought beyond my wildest dreams that I would ever get accepted into a PhD or doctoral program. That's something to say about ambition because that has got to be the only thing that kept me going for all these years. I said that I would never go back to school after I finished my master's but apparently the fire was not quite out yet. When I thought that all was done my ambition relit the fire and kept me going.

If you feel the ambition in you trying to continue, listen to it, believe that it can be done and follow your heart. It takes a lot of heart to get through one of these programs so listen to your heart and go for it if that is what you are feeling.

Reasons

The reasons that someone chooses to consider taking the journey are as original as a person's personality. For every person there is another reason and for every reason, there is probably ten more reasons. We all choose to challenge this level of education for our own personal reason. I'm not going to try to list the many reasons why people make this choice but rather concentrate on why your reason is so important.

The course work isn't likely going to be that hard for someone that has already finished a master's degree. You probably have developed a system that works best for you and have used it to succeed in your studies. So, I'm going to move ahead to the dissertation process and discuss your reason as it pertains to this.

The dissertation process is a long and usually arduous process for most people. It is not intended to be easy or something that can be done in a few weeks. As I have heard, if it was easy everyone would have one. The dissertation process can be very challenging intellectually, emotionally, psychologically, and even some would say physically.

Whatever reason you have chosen to make the journey must be strong enough to keep you going through these hard times. The frustration level can elevate to a point that you would just give up because it seems impossible to get past a certain sticking point. That reason has to be what you fall back on when the going gets tough to give you the motivation to continue.

For me, the reason I started the journey changed probably a few times. What kept me going through the dissertation process was that I didn't want to let my committee chair down. For someone to guide me, stand by me, and motivate me when the going got tough I had no plans to let down. Several times I wanted to just quit and walk away because I became so frustrated with what was happening to me. It seemed like there was no way out at times. My chair was able to say the right words that kept me going without even knowing she was doing that. So, when the times were tough I thought about the sacrifice she was making for me and I didn't want to let her down. I also had a good committee and didn't want to let them down as well. I refer to my chair because you work closely with your chair and they can relate to you more.

While I was in the Navy a mentor once told me that in order to succeed at something you have to want it more than anything in the world. He made it through some of the Navy's toughest special forces training courses so I figured his advice was well worth it. When I started out in the program I made up my mind that I was going to finish no matter what and I wasn't going to let anything stop me. My goal when I started was to finish before my mother closed her eyes. If you can get a good solid reason before you start, one that you know will motivate you then get it and don't let it go. Make a good plan and stick to it. I assure you that you will need it somewhere along the journey, trust me.

When you begin to "hit the wall" as long-distance runners refer to it you have to reply on something to keep you going. You will come to a point that seems like there is no way that you could continue because you have lost focus, burned out, or are simply "spent" and out of gas.

This happens and will likely happen to you along the journey. This is when your reason is desperately needed to pick you up and keep you going. Sometimes you will need to just step away for a while to regain your bearings. During this time your reason has to come front and center to give you the motivation and drive to get back into the race and keep pushing to the finish line or better yet, take the "walk".

CHAPTER FOUR

My Story

As I have mentioned earlier, the journey for me actually started after I had a father to son bonding trip with my oldest son to discuss where he was at in life and what his next move was. I talked about going to school and how much of a commitment that would be. I was practically a cheerleader for a formal college education. Well, the funny thing is I was actually motivating myself to go back to school.

I honestly had no idea what I was getting myself into. No research, no conversations with those that were in a program, or with someone who had finished the program, totally cold. I really didn't know what a dissertation was about or how to write and put one together. I only had a master's degree and the experiences that go with getting through that program. Plus, to top it off I had graduated with my Master's degree 12 years prior to this so I hadn't been in any formal education for 12 years. The odds were stacked against me from the very beginning of ever starting and much less finishing a doctoral program. Within four weeks I was starting classes and on my way on the journey. Filled with enthusiasm and ambition I jumped head first into this program with hopes that I would one day finish.

Knowing what I know now I'd say that I made several big mistakes from the very beginning. Since finances weren't a big factor for me, I didn't have to worry about wasting a lot of money or worry about how I would pay back student loans. If that was a factor from the beginning, I probably would not have taken the journey. A doctoral degree is a big financial undertaking so the decision should not be taken lightly.

After I got into the course work I was pretty comfortable with the assignments and wasn't too over burdened with them. The workload was actually easier to me than when I did my Master's. I did the online track so I had to get used to the way online teaching is done. I can say that after the online experience I don't think I could go back to traditional in the classroom studies. I didn't have any family around to take up my time and was at the full disposal of the time needed to complete the readings and assignments. The reading assignments are very important and I tried to read every single word in order to gain a full understanding of the assignments. This was very time consuming for me. I became accustomed to going to bed at 12 midnight or after while starting at around 6:00 to 6:30 pm every night, 7 days a week. I devoted many hours to my studying and was lucky to not have any distractions other than myself. Again, it is very important to minimize what could distract you because you don't want to fall behind in your studies to any extent.

Once I had taken a few classes I fell into a routine where I was staying after work in my office and doing my homework for up to 5 hours sometimes. I'd take a short 15-minute nap after I was off and then get started on my assignments and readings and stay until 9:00 pm. I did this for about 2-3 years. I spent my weekends usually studying after 5:00 pm on Saturday and Sunday. This went on for about 2-3 years. I had no social life and completely withdrew from any and all social activities other than an occasional birthday party or get together for a special occasion. I put school as my number one priority and didn't let anything get in the way.

During this time I had to purchase a hot spot from my cell phone carrier because I had to keep doing homework while I was on the road or traveling. I would visit my mother back east every year and she didn't have an internet connection or Wi-Fi. This was an unforeseen expense that I incurred and had to maintain while I was in class.

About halfway through the program I started working on my dissertation. We had to attend a residency class at the home campus to get started. This was a very interesting time because you had to choose what you were going to do your research on and begin writing it. We did this through classroom exercises with class participation. This way you got immediate feedback and could hopefully see pass your nose. This process was very eye opening because what you thought from the beginning would work you most likely found out that you still had a lot of time at the drawing board trying to figure it out and convince yourself that this would work.

For me, I changed my plan on what I was going to write about several times. You must be thick-skinned during this phase because what makes sense to you might not make a bit of sense to a trained professional that you are trying to sell your idea to. The instructors in this residency were there to help you understand what you were proposing for your topic. A lot of times I walked away trying to figure out what I was trying to propose too. A thorough understanding of what you are trying to do is needed to successfully negotiate this phase and that isn't always the case. In fact, you really benefit from what they are trying to teach you at this point because you don't want to push on to later find out that you made a wrong turn. I have seen this happen to two friends of mine that are in a doctoral program. Sometimes the foresight doesn't take into account something that might become a problem later on. You could only hope that you meticulously negotiate this process so that you don't have to go back and re-do what you have already done. And believe me this happens more often than not. It's really not like you can avoid it in some cases but a really good look at what you are planning to spend the next few years working on is really worth the time and effort.

As I got deeper and deeper into the dissertation process several other things came to light. You have an idea that you really believe in and really want to see come to fruition. But you have advisors that are called committee members that coach you along the way. Since they have already done the process and have become professionals at how it works they seem to have an eye for what works and what doesn't or can gauge just how hard something will be to work on. Their advice in the process is priceless and can save you a lot of time. My chair told me in our first conversation to not argue with the changes that I get back after I submit my work to them. She told me that I might not agree with something but that the objective is to get done and that I don't necessarily have to agree with everything. It took me some time to grasp this, but she was right. I've had mentors tell me that my dissertation will not look like anything that I started with because of the many re-writes that will take place between starting and finishing. Again, this friend was right. You have to accept that early on or you will likely run into time-consuming disagreements that will cost you in the long run.

I have a saying that I used in a doctoral support group lecture I gave to doctoral candidates that goes like this; you will start out with plans for a car but will end up with a boat. Learn to accept that early on and you will be more successful as you go. Remember that committee members and chairpersons are paid to make corrections and to advise you as you go and many times we don't see it the way they do. That doesn't mean its wrong it just means that it's their advice that you should heed. At the end of the process with a finished dissertation I can honestly say that that was some of the best advice I received because my dissertation turned out to be better that what I originally envisioned.

Another bit of advice that I learned in my journey was to not bite off too much with your plans. At a residency the instructor told us "To not boil the ocean, just a little part of it". You don't want to make your dissertation too big because you are no a pro at this yet and as a novice you might not see just how much work is required for what you want to do. Your idea may not be as practical as you planned from the beginning. Interviewing 50 people might sound easy to do but practically interviewing 50 people could take months because of the transcription and analysis. My plan changed regarding interviews and who I was planning to interview over a lunch date with my cousin and her husband. He suggested that I use a different population and a smaller number of interviewees, and I took that advice and made the change for the better. One of my committee members told me that my research would take forever and that I wasn't qualified to perform it. I scaled down what I was planning and finished a modified version of my plan.

You can have grandiose ideas but must understand how to make your ideas work for you. The advice you receive from committee members is only advice but usually has a lot of validity to it. I stuck to my plan when I was told that it was too much for me to handle but I scaled it down to still meet what I was trying to accomplish. So, as you can see there is some wiggle room but as I mentioned you could end up wasting a lot of time going down the wrong path. It is good to seek wise counsel and heed what you are being told.

Another thing I learned on my journey was to be cognizant of timelines that are required. In order to submit your work at different phases in the process you must meet strict guidelines. The timelines I am speaking to here are directed by the school you attend. The other timelines involved in this process are the ones that we put on ourselves. I've heard doctoral candidates say they would finish at a specific time and become very frustrated and stressed out because they didn't meet that goal. That's a good idea but I suggest that you don't put that stress on yourself and continue to do the work in a timely manner. It was my experience that it took me several years more to finish than I would have liked to but I didn't stress out about it because most of it was out of my hands. When I submitted something, it didn't mean that I was going to get it back when I wanted or thought that I should get it back. The system and committee members' lives have some control of when you get things back. The

IRB process changed while I was submitting, and it took literally 16 months for me to get through IRB. That is unprecedented and probably an oversight on someone's part, but I never let that stress me out or get me down. Had I let that drive me into a stressful situation I probably would never have finished. Sure, it was very frustrating but I never felt that I would let it control me and drive me crazy. Hopefully, that is a onetime event and doesn't happen to you but I wanted to illustrate just how things can happen that you have no control over and hopefully how to deal with them. Committee members also have lives to live and may not return your work when you think they might. Luckily, that wasn't the case with me but I've heard of candidates having this issue.

Another issue that can set you back is the departure of a chair or a committee member. Not all committee members work out the way you want them to. They may drop off your team because of family issues that they need to take care of or just about anything from sickness, death or just don't want to be a committee member anymore. Believe me I've heard some horror stories from colleagues that this happened to. Again, I never had that happen but I did have a committee member drop off my team for personal reasons and it took me about seven months to get a replacement. This set me back another seven months from my perspective finish date, but I didn't let this stress me out or cause me to get off course. These unforeseen things can and will happen so you have to be flexible enough to accept them and to keep on course to finish.

The program calls for you to make certain milestones and requirements to complete your dissertation. These would be a Quality Review Board (QRB), Institutional Review Board (IRB), Quality Review Final (QRF), Oral Defense or some other form of review process depending on the school you are attending. These milestones can take time and sometimes the review yields change that are both good and bad. Good changes are that the review board accepts what you have submitted with few changes, or the review board totally disregards what you have submitted and recommends a different path. I've heard both stories from colleagues and have seen the changes being recommended at residencies. Review boards have produced both exciting moments and devastating moments in a candidate's journey. You must be willing to accept either way it turns out and to keep going regardless of what they tell you. It can be hard to start over again but it is doable. Remember me talking about your plan and how it can be changed as you go along the journey well this is a prime example of that. Having a plan to finish is a good thing but you have to look at the reality of how things play out sometimes in order to not get caught up in self-imposed stress through deadlines you set for yourself.

Another goal that I set for myself was to finish before the hospital I work in moved to a new building and to be able to hang my new degree in my new office. The move date was set for December 2013 and I started in May 2009. Seems like a reasonable goal, four years to finish, right. Well, the move occurred and I was still rolling along on the journey with no projected end date in sight. I finally finished in June of 2016, three years after my first goal. I finally got the opportunity to hang my degree in my new office, three years later. But I never let that stress me out because I knew that I was doing everything I could to complete my dissertation that was in my power. Things happen that you just don't have any control over so you have to let that happen and just keep plugging away.

As you progress through the journey, you meet certain milestones. Each milestone brings about a certain amount of satisfaction and accomplishment. These milestones mark the progress you are making through the maze of requirements presented before you. For me, even though I passed each milestone they all came with a price. When I received word that my QRF was approved there was eight pages of corrections to go along with it. Those corrections had to be reviewed and re-approved before I could move on to the next step. Believe me you become an expert at making corrections after a while.

Nearing the end of my journey, after I was notified that my final QRF was approved it was time to prepare for the oral defense. Actually, for me this was the easiest part because I have been training and teaching for years in the military and in civil service. It was natural for me to speak about something that I felt passionate about and had been working on for so many years.

Finally, the day came for me to do my oral defense and I couldn't wait. Once it was over my chair told me she would call me back in a few minutes to let me know how I did. I sat quietly in the room I did my defense in with the door shut in complete silence waiting for the phone to ring. About ten minutes later the phone rang and it was my chair. She told me that I had done well and congratulated me and called me Dr. Evans. It was the first time that I officially heard that title in front of my name. It meant the world to me to finally reach this goal. I had done it!!

I thanked her and told her how much I appreciated her help and support and that it would not have been possible without her in my corner. When I hung the phone up, I burst into tears, tears of joy that it was finally over. After seven long years I had finally finished.

What I learned

Learning by trial and fire with so much at stake is probably not the best way to enter into something as life changing as the pursuit of a doctoral of PhD degree, but that was the way I chose to do it and luckily for me I was able to accomplish the ultimate goal. Hence, is the reason for why I came up with the idea to write this book? At the core is the idea to help reduce some of the unknowns that someone will come across after they decide to make the journey. The help of a mentor author to provide personal perspectives helps widen the scope of this book and hopefully will appeal to many more people to assist in their personal journey.

In hindsight, one of the first things I learned about this journey was to do your research ahead of time. Get a good idea of what you are getting yourself into before you commit to it. This is a huge commitment as you have seen in the earlier pages, and I can't help to over emphasize that over and over. Know why you want to get started, how you plan to negotiate what you know and be ready for the unexpected to happen, because it will. Also, talk to those that have made the journey to get their perspective and advice. Every little bit helps.

I was told in my first residency that writing a dissertation could likely be a life changing event. It can affect you in many different ways. Getting through this process will make you dig deep into your heart and makeup to figure out what you are about and who you are. This process can try you mentally more than you have ever been tried before. And believe me, being mentally tired can really have an effect on you physically as well. Keeping up with the pace can be demanding considering all the other things you have going on in life along with this. I'd say that it can be very challenging to say the least.

I learned that almost everything I was being told in residencies came true for me. I honestly thought that some of the talk was exaggeration and that it could not really be true, but I learned otherwise and have to say that it all came true. In fact, I could probably walk into a residency now and have a little more to add to what they are already hearing from my own experiences.

I don't tell you all of this to discourage you in any way, but to give you a true perspective of what it is like to pursue a doctorate degree or Ph. D. The advertising that schools do is to get you enrolled and in the program. Before you start the journey, it would be hard to expose you to the reality of the journey and possibly keep you interested in going for it. Also, keep in mind that my experiences are different from someone else's, but I can almost guarantee it that most are somewhat similar in some form or fashion.

Pursuing and achieving a doctorate degree or Ph. D is very rewarding and can open many opportunistic doors to you but there is a rite of passion that you must endure in order to enjoy these opportunities and the satisfaction of accomplishing it.

Another thing I learned from this experience is that it is also very rewarding as you overcome the hurdles that are placed in the journey for you to make progress. Planning for the next checkpoint, working up to it and submitting what's needed is exciting because you put your heart and soul into it and hope for the best. When the day comes that you find out that you succeeded is one of the most exciting and rewarding times, I've had in m my educational journey. Successfully completing a checkpoint helps build confidence it your ability to challenge and overcome that next step. With so many checkpoints on the journey your confidence in yourself is being built up as you go. I've learned to have confidence in what I think, what I do and how I approach things.

Accomplishment is very rewarding and compliments what you put your heart and mind together to produce. This process will definitely reward your hard work with the accomplishments and strides you make.

I've learned to believe in myself regardless of what I am up against. In my undergrad work I was constantly second guessing myself on tests and when writing papers. I always thought that I was a terrible test-taker and that I wasn't smart enough to learn and test well on the topic I was studying. Somewhere in my junior year an instructor took the time to sit down with me and teach me about having the confidence to do what I thought was right and not to ty to appease the teacher or write what I thought the test was looking for. That day I followed his advice and wrote the best test score in the class. That lesson taught me a lot and improved my college experience immensely. Well, I had to revisit that moment in my head to gain the reassurance of what I learned that day and it helped me again as I continued along the journey.

I was presented with situations where either I stuck to my guns or rolled over and gave in to what I was being told. An example of this is when you get back a submission and you think in your heart that you are right and that your committee member is wrong. You must learn to know when to take a stand and when to let it ride and hope for the best. I learned the latter early on for two reasons; my chair suggested it and secondly, because I could stand to learn from it. I bit my tongue more than a few times but in the long run I benefitted from it and was successful because of it. I know of doctoral candidates that have preferred to stand their ground too long and have paid dearly for it with their time and money.

This is a good case of knowing when to put your ego away in a safe place and when to rely on your ego to get you through something. A mentor in my life once told me that there will be times when it is good to be quiet and learn for the situation and to carry on. This advice helped me tremendously as I progressed on my dissertation. In another residency the instructor told us that getting done with your dissertation and graduating is like getting your driver's license. The driver's permit process is the time your spent working on your dissertation. You don't know how to drive yet, that's why you are learning from your committee. Arguing with your committee is like arguing with your driver's license evaluator. They hold the clipboard that says if you can drive or not and if you will be granted a driver's license. When they make a recommendation, you should heed it rather than disagree with it. The committee member holds the same authority through your chair. Learn to follow what they recommend, and you will be successful earlier on than you would be if you chose to argue with them. This was probably the most valuable thing I learned from my chair which shared this with me from our very first meeting. Thank you Dr. V.

CHAPTER FIVE

The Dissertation Process

The dissertation process is a major part of the doctoral journey. Without it the process would not be complete, and the doctoral candidate would not meet the requirements for graduation. By definition a dissertation is a long essay or paper written to meet the requirement for a doctoral degree or Doctor of Philosophy Degree. The specific requirements for a dissertation can and do differ from one college to the next. However, there are many similarities between them. The major that someone is pursuing would dictate the type of dissertation requirements that have to be met. For instance, some schools require a five-chapter dissertation while others only require a four-chapter paper. I believe traditionally the five-chapter is more common among the schools. Along with this requirement is quite a few classes in the curriculum that prepare you for writing the dissertation. Some are basic writing classes and others pertain to the types of methods and research that are part of the requirement to write the dissertation. I would highly recommend that when you take these classes to learn as much as you can because what you don't learn could come back to haunt you and cause you to spend a lot of time relearning during the dissertation process. The method you choose to use is covered in these classes and is an important part, if not the most important part, of your dissertation process. Learn these as thoroughly as you can so that you can explain them and why you choose which one you did for your dissertation. You'll need to know this thoroughly for your oral defense. Much of what you learned in these classes will come into play when you finally are ready to start writing your dissertation.

Another important aspect of writing a dissertation is the use of the American Psychological Association Manual, in short referred to as "APA" manual. This is what is sometimes called the writers bible. The APA manual is used exclusively to format everything written in the dissertation. I strongly advise that if you are required to write a dissertation that you become very familiar with the current edition of the APA manual. I would recommend that you get a copy of it and read it cover to cover paying particular attention to citing references and basic format. There is no arguing with anyone when your paper is not in APA format. Everyone I knew going through the doctoral program had their own personal copy with many earmarked pages throughout the manual. Dissertations commonly end up being from 100 to 200 hundred pages when complete so that's a lot of APA formatting to get right in order to meet the requirement. I can't emphasize enough how important it is to learn the current APA manual and to use it exactly states it. There is no deviation from the APA in any form or fashion. Once you get to the writing phase, the APA will become a perpetual writing companion and should be referred to as often as needed.

With all of that said about the importance of the APA manual there is one aspect that you should be familiar with. The APA manual is updated from time to time and if by chance you are in the process of writing your dissertation you will likely have to convert to the updated version which might mean that you will have some additional editing to do to meet the requirements for the newer version. This happened to me and to many other colleges of mine that were writing their dissertations at the same time. Luckily there wasn't that much that changed so the editing didn't take too long, but it was just another step added to an already long process. This is one reason that you want to finish your dissertation as soon as you can.

It is common practice to get burned out in the dissertation process and prolong finishing it or literally just stop writing it all together. There are many speed bumps in this process that will try your patience, not to mention life's natural occurrences itself.

Before you start to put pen to paper or spend hours in front of a computer you must come up with a topic that you want to write about. This topic must meet several requirements and pass a review and acceptance by the school before you start writing. This is not an easy task by any means. What I found out about this is that you must be passionate about your topic and one that you are truly interested in writing about. I have a saying about the topic you come up with and the end result of your dissertation that goes like this, you start out with plans for a car and end up with making a boat. It never starts and ends the same. I changed my idea several times before I finally came up with my final topic. In fact, my final topic came up at a luncheon I was at having a conversation with a family member that suggested how to narrow my audience down to a specific group. As a result of the conversation my final change to my topic was formed and I went on to finish my dissertation. So, you never know when it will hit but I guarantee that it won't be the first thing you come up with. Let your creative juices flow when you are coming up with a topic and don't limit yourself to your first idea. Also, I had several people tell me that my topic wasn't good enough to write about, but I stuck to my guns and continued to push through with my idea and wrote and finished my dissertation with that topic. Be open with what people tell you as you formulate your topic but follow your gut feeling because it's your paper and you are the author.

School advisors will help steer you in the right direction, based on their previous experiences so take their advice wisely.

After you come up with a starting idea you will then have to enlist a committee to help you along the journey. You will first find a chairperson, commonly referred to as the "chair" and most likely two committee members. The school you go to will assist you in this process. This committee's purpose is to review your work step by step and make recommendations to you along the way. The key to getting a good chair is that they have to be interested in the topic you picked and be familiar with the method that you choose to use for your dissertation. This is an invaluable part of the process. You don't want a chair or committee member that is unfamiliar with your method once you get started. The committee is there to assist you, but at times will drive you crazy because they don't always make the same recommendations. Also, along the Journey you will submit to your committee what you have written so far and get it back several days later with many corrections from each committee member. It can be mind-blowing and drive you crazy trying to figure out what they are saying and then making the corrections. I must have made 500 or more corrections along the way. I once worked with a colleague that told me that she flat out refused to make any more corrections on her final draft after it came back for the 30th time. This process definitely has its ups and downs. The best advice I can give you here is to learn to accept criticism from your committee, and more especially from your chair. Their criticism at times may sound personal but in reality, it is not and is for your own good. Remember, they have already been through the process and are there to help you get through it. Their criticism may save you a lot of time and effort in the future as you get further along into the process.

When I wrote my dissertation, I was required to write a five-chapter version as required by my school. The five chapters were #1 Introduction, #2 Literature Review, #3 Methodology, #4 Presentation of Research, and #5 Conclusion and Summary. These are the basic 5 chapters that make up the dissertation. They may have different but similar titles but are relatively the same. Each chapter will have a rubric or guide to use to ensure that you cover all of the requirements relatively the same. Each chapter should be between about 20-30 pages. As you can see the number of pages starts to add up as you write. My dissertation ended up being 136 pages long. I have friends that were in school with me that wrote nearly 100 for their first 3 chapters. In my opinion that is too long. Your chair should be your guide to help you determine how long your chapters should be. My advice here is to write what you need to write and try not to write too much. Learn to be succinct in your writing and get to the point with what you are trying to convey. Being too wordy can actually work against you when trying to stick to the strict requirements of the dissertation. Another saying we had in school about this is, "don't try to boil the sea, just get a cup of water and boil it". Sometimes you can bite off too much in a topic and chapter and end up writing way too much than you need to. You have to remember to make your point and to move on.

The mid dissertation requirement that needs to be met is to get approval to conduct research from the Institutional Review Board or IRB. The approval of the IRB is critical and pertinent in order to conduct your research. This is an ethical review of your proposed research method and how you plan to conduct your research. If humans are involved, i.e., surveys or interviews, the IRB must review your plan to ensure that no human rights are violated and that all your research is conducted in an ethical manner. This process usually takes about 2 weeks to a month depending on when you submit your proposal. Learn what the IRB is looking for to avoid any problems when you submit your proposal.

I didn't experience this, but I have seen in recent years some schools have added additional requirements that you must pass an oral defense of your first 3 chapters (proposal) before you can begin conducting your research and that you must submit your methodology to a board for review and approval concurrently with your IRB submission.

The dissertation process can take several years to complete. There's no shame in taking your time and doing a good job. This is not a race, it's a journey. With that said, let me emphasize a point that you need to keep in mind while working on your dissertation. Time can become an issue with the content of the dissertation because in chapter 2 the references you use should not be more than 5 years old. You're likely going to have a few references that are 5 years old or older, but the majority must be less than 5 years old. This can present a problem if you start and for some reason have to stop for a year or two due to unforeseen circumstances. Sickness, family illness, change of employment are a few of the issues that could come up while you are writing your dissertation that can present a problem for you. A way to hopefully prevent this from becoming a big problem is to work on your dissertation every day. Do a little at a time but don't stop all together. I was given the advice to work on it for at least 15 minutes a day no matter how I felt about it. Some days you can work for hours if you are in the flow and some days, you'll be good if you can get those 15 minutes out. You will experience what is sometimes called "writer's block", which is a term that describes when your writing creativity is just not there, and you have no desire to work on a paper. You'll likely learn to recognize this and know when to just do a little on that day. Sometimes you will just have to put it away for a few days to clear your mind and come back when you feel fresh. The main point is to not give up and get lazy during this process. It is a long and hard process by design and you'll just have to stick it out to get through it.

Once you finally get all of your chapters written and finally approved by your committee the last requirement will be to do an oral defense of your dissertation. This is usually a PowerPoint presentation of your dissertation. Using somewhere between 20 and 30 slides you will be required present your dissertation to a committee, usually your committee, to show your work and take them through all 5 chapters concluding with what your research accomplished or what you found out from your research. Your research is done to determine through methodology if the conclusion is what you expected or what you learned from it. In my dissertation I came up with results that weren't expected which caused a problem at first until I could write about and explain what I found out. It was interesting to me since my research showed positive results to the problem I picked as a topic. The fascinating thing to me about the research is that you really never know what you are going to come up with until all the work is done.

CHAPTER SIX

Motivation and Advice

Motivation for a program like a PhD or a doctoral degree must come from inside an individual. You must have that desire to succeed and something to push you when times are tough. For this I'd like to share a short "sea story" of something that happened to me during my naval career. I was attending a six-month school for preventive medicine and the director was greeting our class on the first day. His words to us for motivational guidance to the class were "priority and persistence". He said that you have to first set your priority and then you must persist to meet it. He was right, I took these words of wisdom to heart from the first time I heard them and have used them ever since. I have used them through all of my degree work and have succeeded because of them.

Over time I have added one more word to this and that being "time". It takes time to succeed at something that is worthwhile to achieve. Factor in the time that it will take for you to have this priority and persistence and you will come up with your own recipe for success. I used to talk to my sons about time and how it plays such an important part in your success. You must learn to respect time and how to manage it to your benefit. I told my sons when they were growing up an example of this is when a farmer plants a crop for profit. First, he must prepare the soil, then plant the seed, water and care for it, and finally harvest it. Crops take time for them to be suitable for sale and profit. Any mismanagement of time with a crop can easily end up as a disaster and be nonprofitable to the farmer, therefore time well spent will have a good yield, but time not spent well will not result in a product.

Accomplishing a PhD or doctoral degree takes anywhere from four to eight years, depending on some controllable and noncontrollable factors. During this period there will be times that you will need to draw from your source of motivation to enable you to make it through the tough times. For me, I wanted to give up many times but for whatever reason kept on going and hoping that one day I would finally finish this. I drew strength from my motivation, continuously telling myself that I was going to finish if I stayed on track and listened to my heart. I knew that someday it would all come together. I set my priority of doing some work on my dissertation every day, no matter if it was only 15 minutes or several hours, at least it would be some progress. I didn't want time to get away from me by looking at the calendar one day and realizing that I just missed an opportunity over the past few months to get something done. So, I did my best to not let time get away from me. Respect time and time will respect you.

Setting the priority is easier said than done. I persevered by making it my goal to accomplish something every day regardless of how I felt when I sat down to do some writing. I would usually have to be in the mood to write and that took some time even though my intent was to start as soon as I sat down. I would get in front of the computer at 7:00 pm but not really get started until 8:00 pm. I would surf the net or get distracted with something else. Once I started working on my dissertation I had to change that and start writing as soon as I sat down in order to get something done. That was hard to do but a necessary change in order to make progress.

So, make it a **PRIORITY** in your everyday life, **PERSEVERE** by doing something every day and don't let **TIME** get away from you by not utilizing it wisely. As time went on, I fell into a groove that worked well for me and I persisted on the things that I had control over. Remember that I mentioned that there are things that you will not have control over as you go along the journey. You have to learn to accept those moments and embrace the time that you do have control over. Don't let there be a lag in time because of something that you can't get done because there will be those moments as well.

You can't get time back once it's gone so you must always use it to your advantage.

A Motivational Tool – The TAN Philosophy

Throughout my naval career I had the opportunity to connect with a lot of people that were ambitious and had a plan to get ahead in life. Many were motivated to go to school to further their education and increase their opportunity to become a commissioned officer. Others were motivated to rise up through the ranks and achieve the highest rank they possibly could. During this time, I had the opportunity to meet and mentor some sailors that went on to have great careers and made a difference for their families and communities. I was fortunate and blessed enough to have a great set of mentors guide me as I progressed through my career as well. Mentors would serendipitously appear at phases of my life where they offered advice that changed my life in constructive and positive ways. At one time an unsuspecting mentor advised me to change my major while I was working on my bachelor's degree. He couldn't have been timelier or offer any better advice at that time in my education. I made the change and the timing worked out perfectly and I finished with literally five days left before I was due to transfer.

I met a friend during one of my tours of duty that became the one mentor that helped guide me to the success

I enjoy today by instilling in me a sense of confidence that I didn't have. During one of my darkest times he helped me believe in myself and overcome the issues that put me in that dark mindset. Still to this day I hear from him almost daily in email and from time to time talk on the phone. I tell you this story because after meeting him I came up with what I call the TAN Philosophy. This is not a scientific formula or philosophy that you will find in a textbook. I gave it this name because of the first letters of what TAN stands for. I have shared this with many people over the years. Some even have a framed version of this hanging on their I love me wall. I planned many years ago to sit down and write a book about this but never got around to it. So, since it is a form of motivation, I will share it with you in this book.

The TAN philosophy is a motivational tool to keep you on the right track when your mind is telling you to do something different. It can be applied to other areas of your life other than keeping you motivated to keep going while in school. I originally used it to teach people to keep going when times got hard. I encouraged them to refer to it as a tool to keep them on track.

So, here it is.

"T" is for - Take a negative thing and turn it positive
"A" is for – Always stay a step ahead
"N" is for – Never let them see you sweat but let them know when you're mad.

Let me explain what each letter means in context.

T is for "Take a negative thing and turn is positive" is a way of looking at something when the face value of something is negative. Take for example you have something that happens to you that makes you mad enough to say something or do something that you would regret later. You get mad at something your boss says to you and you respond by saying something negative bordering on disrespect. This could have some negative consequences if you say what's on your mind or what is not appropriate at the wrong time. Instead, you could respond by not saying anything and walking away. You could use that negative energy to go to the gym with you and push yourself to perform better than you usually do. In my twenties and thirties, I lifted weights at the gym three days a week. When I got mad about something I would use that negative energy to fuel my drive at the gym and lift more weight or do more sets. On a normal day I couldn't do that because I was out of energy. But when I was mad about something I could use that to have a better day at the gym. When I used to run long distances, I would use that anger to channel what I was thinking on a long run and not be so worried about how I felt physically while I was running. I would find that I ran better when something was bothering me than I did on a day that my mind was clear. So, this is how I channeled a negative thing and turned it positive. Believe me, I learned this through experience and over time. As I got older, I learned to use this to my benefit and not make a bad situation worse than it was.

So how does this apply to the doctoral journey? Well, remember me talking about my experience in first grade coming home with B's on my report card. Well, that somehow motivated me to keep pushing my way through school because it left a negative impression on me that lasted well into my adult years. That negative impression motivated me to continue through my schooling and to achieve the highest level possible that I could. Remember I also mentioned earlier that my doctoral goal was to finish before my mother closed her eyes for good, well that was also a strong motivation for me to continue when things got hard to continue when I couldn't see the light. Sometimes I wonder if I hadn't had something negative happen to me at that early age would I have had the drive and motivation to continue my education all the way up to a doctoral degree. This goes to show that tough love isn't always a bad thing and that you might not be actually hurting someone that you are using it on.

Another negative incidence that happened in my naval career took place in a small office where I fell out of grace with my leadership and said something that got me into trouble with my boss. I was almost fired from my current job because of it and it caused a lot of problems for me. At the advice of my mentor, I was able to defuse the situation and in time turn it around in a positive direction. It took some time but as a result I was nominated for and received the highest award in the command for the work I did following this incident. I was able to take this very negative incident and use it to fuel my positive actions in my favor and turn the whole situation around. I hadn't come up with the TAN philosophy yet but learned from my mentor how to carry myself following a negative situation.

The object here is not to wait until something negative happens to try this out and see if it works for you but to be prepared with a game plan on how to respond to something like this on the event that it happens. It's not so easy to turn things around when something negative happens but being able to do it can save a lot of heartburn and turn things in the right direction.

So, this applies to each and every one of us that experiences something negative in their lives that they have to deal with. I believe that pretty much includes all of us in some form or fashion. Take a negative event in your life and turn it positive by giving yourself more energy to tackle an assignment in school or to put more time into your dissertation work than you would normally do.

When you work on your dissertation you will find that there will be times when you receive recommendations and corrections from three people, your chair and your committee, that may contradict each other but you have to figure out what the best recommendation is, fix it and resubmit it. This can be very perplexing and drive a perfectionist crazy. It's not easy to come up with the right solution that will make all three happy at the same time. This can create a stressful situation and leave you very confused at times. This negative can be turned positive by taking your time and doing some thorough research to turn it around and giving yourself time to make the corrections. Use this negative energy to learn why it is to be corrected and make a workable change to meet the recommendation. This will not always happen like this, so I encourage you to adapt as quickly as you can to this so that the negative energy doesn't derail you. And believe me it can and has derailed me and some of the best of us.

In the workplace learn to take a negative thing and turn it positive because too many negatives can have a detrimental effect on your livelihood if they happen to fast and too many. People say things to the wrong person when they are mad about a decision or task that happens to them while at work. This is where I first applied this philosophy to and it has helped me and many people over the years.

A is for "Always stay a step ahead" is a way of how to deal with the known things that happen to you. Originally, this was meant to anticipate what your boss was planning and stay out in front of them so that you don't fall behind the eight ball. If you know what is coming up or next plan to meet that demand before it happens and satisfy the boss before they ask for something.

I used to inspect navy ships environmental health programs at one of my duty stations and the ships that did the best were the ones that had everything out that I was inspecting before I got there so I didn't have to ask for anything. The ships that did poorly were the ones that weren't ready for the inspection and had nothing out for my review. So, I learned from this that if you stay ahead of what is going to happen then leadership didn't ask too many questions and stayed satisfied more often than not. That generally makes my day when I must deal less with what should have been done rather than being behind the eight ball and playing catch up. Staying a step ahead keeps all those concerned in a better place than if someone has to constantly tell you what you need to be doing.

So, how does this apply to the doctoral journey? While you are in the didactic phase it's pretty much self-explanatory. You have an assignment to do and a date that it is due, so you know what you have to do. The problem here is that many of us are natural procrastinators and will put off an assignment until the last minute. I can honestly say that I did my best work when my back was against the wall and I was behind the eight ball. Not a good place to be and can have negative consequences if allowed to continue throughout your degree.

So, I began to use this and stay ahead of my assignments and it paid dividends when I got to the dissertation phase because I learned to make a plan and to stick to it. The dissertation process can and will trip you up somewhere along the way regardless of how well you plan it. But, you can reduce the issues if you plan for them and try your best to stay out ahead of them. Believe me, easier said than done but at least I had a plan. Some of the process is hard to plan ahead for but whatever you perceive that can be planned for by all means plan for it and stay out ahead of it.

This applies in life as well. In the workplace if you know what the boss is looking for make their job easier and get it done ahead of time. Managing someone that gets the job done is much easier than managing someone that doesn't. During my years in the navy and working after I retired I've seen people fed up with things that they had control over. I've seen them mad or angry about the way that things were going. Many times, it was their own fault and they failed to plan ahead for the upcoming task or event. I would tell them that if you know something is due than do it and get it out of the way. Some honestly couldn't see that until we had a talk about it and it began to make sense to them. It's almost like putting oil in your car. If the oil light comes on don't wait two more weeks before you get your oil changed. Get it changed as soon as the light comes on to avoid any engine problems that may stem from that situation.

N is for "Never let them see you sweat but let them know when you are mad".

This is an interesting one for a student because you have to be careful of what you get mad about and weigh the consequences that may be the result of you letting your faculty know about it.

Let me begin with an example for this one that happened to me. During my dissertation phase I seemed to hit all the hurdles when I was submitting to the Institutional Review Board (IRB). What should have taken sixteen days took sixteen months, literally. I'm not badmouthing anyone or any system but merely stating what happened to me.

After literally about a year of going back and forth with this submission I finally got upset that it was taking so long and decided to contact the school through my chair. The result was several emails going back and forth about why I was stuck in the process. Now I don't encourage or endorse this but there comes a time when you have to speak up if things are just way off course. This was one of those situations. I tried my best to not use this route but eventually had to. I can say that I got results and the process was jump started and I continued with the journey.

If you are one that gets upset a lot and lets them see you sweat, so to say, then you might not get the results you need when the time comes to show them you are mad. It's kind of like crying wolf in a sense. As the moral of that story goes, don't use the horn until you absolutely have to. Don't let them know you are mad until you absolutely have to otherwise you will burn up your chances of getting something done.

I have also seen doctoral candidates get very upset with their chairs and argue point after point with them again, using that horn too much decreases your chances of having it when you really need it. My chair told me when we first met to argue less and do more. The object is to get through the process and finish and then make things your way. She was right. The less I learned to object to corrections or recommendations the faster the pace was and the closer I got to finishing. Something to know here is that the chair controls your progress, not you. So, get along with your chair unless you absolutely have to let them know that you are mad. Be prepared to deal with the consequences if there is a bad turnout due to the situation.

So, what's motivating about the "N"? The motivating thing here is to tell yourself to deal with what is in front of you as best you can. Dealing with the issues gets you closer to finishing than if you don't deal with them in a favorable way. No, I'm not telling you to give in to everything but more to pick your battles before you engage. Too many battles can derail you for more time and more time can work against you staying in the program. Candidates get discouraged with the process and work themselves into a state of anger that results in taking longer and possibly losing motivation to continue, hence the high ABD rate. There are a lot of ABD candidates that got frustrated with the process along the way and just never finished. Occasionally I run into one of them from time to time and try to talk them into getting back into the swing of things.

The dissertation process is designed to be tough and sometimes unrelenting. That's the challenge of it, to see if you have what it takes to complete it. Remember I said early on that it was designed to be hard or everyone would have a PhD or doctorate degree. They are hard to obtain for a purpose. The institutions that have doctoral programs have no plan to make it any easier for you to complete a doctoral program so keep that in mind while you are on the doctoral journey.

"I Can"

Another motivator that I would like to share with you one that has helped me with many of the challenges that I have faced in my personal life and that is simply saying "I can". Whenever you venture into something that seems foreign to you or something that you just don't think you can do your mind plays a game with you telling you that you can't do something. You set a goal based on evidence that someone else did what you want to but for some reason you just feel that it is out of your grasp and can't be done.

For instance, you take up running as a way to improve and maintain your health. Along with this you begin to really enjoy running and become comfortable with it. Next thing you know you are setting goals for yourself and one that you set for running is to break the 6-minute mile barrier someday. You're running 7-minute miles now and feel that someday you will be able to make the 6:30 and then the 6:00 minute mile. After trying to improve your time after a while you hit a wall or plateau that you just can't get past no matter how hard you try. Your mind starts telling you that you can't achieve that goal no manner what you do. At this point your mind starts working against you and you can't get it out of your head.

The "I can't" bug begins to eat away at your desire and ambition to achieve that seemingly hard to achieve or near impossible goal you have set for yourself, and you begin to give up on that goal. Once that "I can't" frame of mind begins to set in it can take away the positive attitude you once had about achieving that goal. This happens more than imagined with doctoral and PhD candidates because of the hurdles on the journey. Sometimes they seem to be unconquerable and unachievable at times. This is where the "I can" mindset has to kick in and push the negativity out of your head. There are probably a large number ABD's out there that have never finished because the "I can't" bug bit them. I have come across two people that fit that category in my travels. That is something many are not proud of but will tell you if you can recognize it. My best guess is that they were seeking some motivation for getting back in the program when they revealed to me their ABD status and why they were in this situation.

When this scenario begins to unravel in your journey you need to be able to quickly recognize the symptoms and tell yourself that you are not going to let this happen to you. You set a goal and you will achieve it no matter what they throw at you. You will run that 6-minute mile no matter how hard it gets for you.

Let me share another scenario with you. My favorite hobby is flying radio-controlled helicopters when I get the time. The problem with that statement is that you must make time and lots of it if you plan to get good at it. RC helicopters are expensive and to repair them after a crash can be very expensive as well. So, you have to make time to fly them as often as you can to eventually get good at it. Right now, I would consider myself an advanced novice with a lot more to learn. I can hold my own but there is a steep learning curve and I am just beginning to climb the upside of the curve.

Recently, I was out flying, and the wind had picked up and I got a little nervous to go fly in it because the wind can play tricks on you and take control of the helicopter and make it hard to control. Other pilots had been out flying it in but with much more experience than me. As I voiced my concern about flying in the wind a fellow pilot told me to think positive. He told me that it was all in my head and that I could fly in the wind with no problem. I followed his advice and went out and flew my helicopter and luck fully I was able to control it and build my confidence at the same time. He showed me that I could fly in it if I believed I could and not have any negative thoughts about what could happen. I put in my head that "I can" do this and followed my thoughts and feelings and was able to accomplish my goal of flying that day. That one event helped me to build my confidence in flying when the wind had a little kick to it.

This reminded me of when I was working on my dissertation because there was a many-a-day when I felt that I would never finish this, but I replaced those thoughts with "I can" and was able to keep pushing on through it. You have to believe in yourself and your ability to keep going when the odds are stacked against you. On the journey you will find many days when it will be hard to keep going but you set the goal and only you can achieve it. Motivating yourself to keep going has to come from you, how you perceive things and how you can turn them into positive thoughts about why you should keep going.

For a long time, I've always thought of the negatives of flying. A $500-dollar helicopter could crash and cost you $100 dollars to fix. So, I would always have it in the back of my mind that I could and probably would crash if I flew in any conditions other than no wind at all.

Repairing RC helicopters can get expensive if you crash a lot. We have a saying in the RC helicopter world and that is "it's not a matter of if you are going to crash, but more of a matter of when you will crash". The learning curve is steep, and you will crash one of these days, so you better accept it when you start out in the hobby, or you won't be flying for long.

The odds are against you that you will become an expert pilot overnight unless you are a child prodigy and can just grasp the sport by both horns from the beginning. Very few young pilots have entered the sport and done well early on but that number can be counted on one hand'.

Chances are you are not going to grasp the dissertation process early on and just breeze through it unscathed. Very few have been able to I'm sure, but I have never met any of them yet. You have to accept early on that the journey will be a rough one and keep a positive mindset to succeed. I've gotten better with my skills for flying over time because I've accepted that I will someday crash and to not be fearful of flying because of that possibility. When you only fly on weekends your skills don't get much better than they were last week. Your ability to do something better doesn't get much better week to week because of your fear of crashing if you get out of your comfort zone. So, you stay in your comfort zone and it takes a long time before you actually get any better. The pro's do it every day until they get really good.

A really good pilot told me that he flew almost every day for three years to get to the level of skill that he was at. I bring this up because the same principle applies to the dissertation process. You have to attack it every day to build you skills and confidence to get through it. The more you are familiar with it the better you will express it on paper and the more you will succeed at it. I began flying every day at lunchtime at work and my skills got better pretty quick. I was able to control the helicopter much better and was building my confidence to a level that I got rid of my nervousness about crashing and flew with confidence. I really felt the difference in about a three-month time period.

This is the same experience I had while working on my dissertation. My chair and other mentors told me to work on it every day no matter how I felt. I had a hard time putting this into action but eventually I was able to make this happen. By pushing myself and telling myself that "I can" I was able to continue pushing on through the hard spots and continue making progress. Believe me, this isn't or wasn't easy but as time went on and I kept pushing myself in this direction it became easier and eventually the norm for me. You can also do this if you put your mind to it and push yourself in this direction.

Like A New Lifestyle

Changing your habits to be successful writing a dissertation is similar to beginning a new lifestyle of eating healthier. First, something brings you to the conclusion that you have to make a change for a healthier lifestyle.

This could be either lose and control your weight or to eat healthier to control a disease process. Let's just say it is for your weight. Next, you must put down and stop eating the junk food you've come to love so much and then replace it with healthier choices that at first don't taste nearly as good in the beginning. If you approach this change slowly and don't try to force it in a short time period, you will eventually be successful at changing your lifestyle. Stop eating the amount of junk food you eat in a day to a lesser amount in a day. Then stop eating junk food every day and only eat it every other day. Eventually, you can decide to stop eating it all together and that makes it easier to cut it out of your diet over time. This is a step in the right direction of achieving the goal of eating healthier foods for weight control.

This same principle can be applied to chipping away at your dissertation. You already know what the ultimate goal is, so you can plan to chip away at it systematically over time. Make a plan that is simple for you to stay with and follow it religiously. Like the ole' saying goes, "how do you eat an elephant, one piece at a time". How do you complete a dissertation, one sentence at a time?

A dissertation is something that you don't normally do in life so changing your lifestyle to adapt to accomplishing this goal takes some work. You must make the change slowly and deliberately and stick to the plan in order for it to work.

The dissertation process is designed to take a long time. There are certain objectives that are built into the process to ensure that you learn the how's, the why's, the when's, and to become good at it. Writing a dissertation isn't something that can be done overnight. By going back and forth many times with your committee with rewrites and new material you will learn the objectives through doing it and not just reading and memorizing things.

Let me expound on the changing lifestyle thought some more. The process of writing a dissertation is partly, if not a majority, done to transform you into becoming a scholar in your own right. Dissertations are scholarly work because of the way that are researched and written. In the process you are transformed from someone who has written many papers in your undergrad and graduate work to the author of a research paper with a great deal of depth. This didn't happen in a vacuum or overnight. It took a lot of time and effort to get to this point. You most likely took a lot of classes and wrote a lot of papers to get to the level of writing to write a dissertation.

During this process (previous degree work) you had and used some form of motivation to keep you going to finally reach your goal. This motivation might have been short lived or something that you continued to come back to time and time again because it worked. Whatever it was it helped work for you and likely changed something in your life to make it to that end.

This form of motivation can be counted on again to get you through a doctoral or PhD program. Keep in mind that this is a different type of writing than you are probably used to and that it takes a lot more time to finish. Therefore, you will need a form of motivation that can stand the test of time and continue to motivate you for a longer period of time.

Changing a lifestyle takes time and requires you to keep yourself motivated in order to accomplish your goal. People set themselves up on a diet and many times for one reason or another "fall off the wagon" and never achieve their goal. This could be due to losing their motivation to continue and ending up stopping and gaining the weight back.

Another example of a lifestyle change that I have seen that takes an enormous amount of time and motivation to complete is tobacco cessation. Quitting the use of tobacco, either smoking or smokeless tobacco, is a hard process to enter into and to complete. To make a change like that takes a lot of motivation and a focus on the end goal that can't be shaken. From my experience working around people that are trying to quit smoking I have seen that it isn't easy by any stretch of the imagination. People really have to work hard at it and stay focused on their goal in order to achieve it.

Quitting smoking can have a physical as well as a psychological effect on someone. Regardless, they have to know what the goal is, prioritize it, keep focused and preserve to get to it. There has to be a certain degree of motivation that keeps them going when they just want to give in and have that cigarette or chew.

Pursuing a doctoral degree or PhD can have the same effect on you. Physically, it can get pretty tiresome staying up late nights working on your dissertation when you have to go to work the next day. You stay up night after night because you are driven to finish this goal. It can and does wear you out from time to time because your body is not wired this way and it takes a toll on you. Psychologically, it can have an effect on you as well for several reasons. You might be used to getting instant or short termed gratification from writing papers in your earlier work as you progressed through your degrees. Well, most likely it won't be the same for the dissertation due to the nature of how a portion is submitted and reviewed by your committee. They may take a few days or more than a week to return the portion back to you with many recommended corrections. In your mind you didn't see this coming but must deal with it once you get it back. This can have a tough psychological effect on your ego, your confidence, or your self-esteem.

These effects chew away at you and can steal your motivation if you are not careful. You have to be aware of this and learn how to identify the signs and symptoms of this before they get the best of you. There is always something that is going to stir your mind away from your ultimate goal. That negative thought can grow large enough that it steals your desire to finish and stops you from accomplishing your goal. By knowing what that negative feeling is can help you stop it before it starts.

My way of keeping myself motivated throughout the journey was to be aware of the negative things and to turn them off as soon as I saw them coming. Some of these negative things for me were the many corrections from my committee, the time delay of getting through the IRB submission process, changing my topic several times until I got it right, changing the method I was planning to use several times and simply taking so long to finish. Every time I felt a negative thought I turned it off by telling myself not to worry about it, to just keep going. I told myself many times to not give in and give up, that that was what they wanted me to do. They being the system, not an individual. The truth be known, I wanted to give up and walk away many times but for some reason just kept going.

At one point after I finally finished all five chapters of my dissertation but hadn't had it reviewed by my committee in its entirety, I wanted to quit, telling myself that I wrote all five chapters and that that was good enough for me. But for some reason I kept going and telling myself that it wasn't completed yet and that I wasn't going to waste this much time, effort, and money and not get what I came for. I couldn't live with the idea in my head that I started a program but never finished it, so that motivated me to keep going regardless of how I felt about it at that particular moment. That motivation carried with me throughout the seven years it took me to finish my doctorate.

It wasn't easy and I'm sure that nobody that has one will tell you that it was easy but that is what makes it so worthwhile to go after it and achieve it. Finally seeing the light at the end of the tunnel after my final review and heading into my oral defense was a strong confirmation that I was finally going to finish. After I finished my oral defense and my chair called me back ten minutes later and called me Doctor Evans I knew that all of my efforts had finally paid off. Honestly, I broke out crying tears of joy that it was finally over, that I had achieved my ultimate goal. Finishing reinforced in me that I can do anything that I put my mind to and that all of the motivation that I used worked as planned.

Finishing my doctorate degree was the hardest challenge that I have ever faced in my life. It was also the biggest accomplishment that I achieved in my life. Nobody handed it to me, I had to work very hard to get it. Finishing this degree was a test of my intellect, my patience, my ability to stay on the course and finally a test of who I am. I stayed true to myself and believed that if I gave it everything I had that I could not be denied from achieving my goal.

Before and After

In this last section, I'm going to talk about what your before you started the program expectations were and what your after you finish the program results are. I'm also going to add in some hindsight Monday Morning Quarterbacking that we all do to second guess ourselves. Obviously if you are reading this book for advice, you haven't started anything yet, so I am going to talk exclusively about my experience with this. The earlier chapters in this book are aimed at helping you decide if this program is for you. This section is my perspective on that matter. Keep in mind that we all have a different perspective, therefore you may agree or disagree with my personal perspective.

I talked about age earlier in the book as being a factor that could weigh into the decision process for starting a course like this. I was 52 years old when I started with most of my career in the rearview mirror. As I mentioned earlier, I challenged this program for personal reasons, mainly to see if I could make it through it. With the GI Bill, I had financial support along the way so that I wouldn't go bankrupt trying to pay for this program. I honestly didn't have many expectations when I started. I really didn't do the research I should have but knew it wasn't going to be easy. The only other expectation I had was that I knew I wanted to teach college at some level in the future and knew a doctoral level degree would help get me there. I was well aware that in my present career it wouldn't change anything except the nameplate on my office door. Several people where I worked thought that the next level degree would warrant a pay raise for the level of education that a doctoral is at. The truth of the matter is that it had no bearing on my position description therefore wasn't required to do my job. A position description spells out what degree is required for the position and a doctorate was not required when I got hired about 4 years prior to starting this job. I later found out that several of the people I worked around had doctorates but weren't hired for their educational level as well and didn't use the title "Dr." in their professional correspondence. So, if your motivation for this type of program is to beef up your resume for a doctoral level job make sure that the position description for the job calls for a doctorate degree so that you get paid for having it.

I honestly didn't have many expectations before starting the program. I kind of went into it blindly and reacted to whatever was expected of me. In a way I think that was to my benefit since it didn't conflict with anything I brought to the program with me. I realized quickly that the structure of this program was very different with what I was used to and that I had to also adapt to an online educational environment. I didn't think I would adapt at first because I thought I needed the classroom environment to learn but I found out that I really liked the online education method better and would prefer it in the future. It took about 2-3 classes to get used to it but once I did it was smooth sailing after that.

After I finished the program, I took a break from academia to catch my breath and get used to not working on my dissertation. I needed the break bad because working on the dissertation really changes your life in terms of how you spend your time. Getting back to something normal was important to me so I took the time to do so.

As I mentioned earlier, having a doctorate degree had no effect on my current employment. I was well aware of that from the beginning. I still had an interest in teaching, so I reached out to several universities and inquired about teaching jobs. I didn't get the response that I thought I would in the beginning and must honestly say that I began to lose interest in teaching because of all of the requirements that I saw that the colleges required. It meant that I would have to do more required courses and qualifications that I wasn't particularly crazy about doing. Plus, I was close to retiring from my current job and wasn't interested in doing any mandatory or required classwork. I realized for myself that age had now played an important part in my "after" experience of post-doctorate experience. I had worked for the government for 45 years, 30 active duty in the Navy and 15 with Civil Service. I was tired of a structured world and just wanted to experience the retired life for a bit. I needed to decompress and put the working world behind me now.

My "after" post-doctorate experience just took another unexpected turn. At this point its probably best to say that I am not a good example of what to do with your doctorate degree after you graduate. There are many opportunities out there available that a doctorate degree can open a door to. I would encourage a new perspective doctoral candidate to explore the post-doctorate possibilities before they start a program to have an idea and a goal to work towards and to motivate them when the going gets tough. I'm sure that if I really put my heart into it I could have found something post-doctorate to make the journey more worthwhile but didn't put the effort into it. The important message to take away from this section is that you have some sort of plan or goal to work towards after you finish your degree. Doctoral degrees open many doors so take full advantage of the opportunities that your efforts have provided for you.

CHAPTER SEVEN

Post-Doctoral Degree Advice

Now let me talk to you about the post-doctoral (or PhD) phase of this program. Keep in mind that I have only had my doctoral degree for two years at the writing of this book, but I have learned a lot from my colleagues that have doctorates in this short time.

A mentor and friend from my work that has a doctorate degree joked with me about what I will likely do after I graduate. She said that I would want to put "Dr." on everything, business cards, desk nameplates and office nameplates and probably a lot of other things. She said that that was ok but to not go overboard. She was right to an extent. I made new business cards, a nameplate for my office and a stamp for paperwork that I routinely do that requires a printed name or stamp. I considered these as things that I had to do for my job. But I stopped there. I didn't tell people to call me "Dr."

and didn't even mention it unless it was pertinent to what I was doing.

A colleague that has a PhD once told me that the reason why the dissertation takes so long is because they purposely beat you down and wear you out to teach you to be humble and not egotistical when you get your degree. She said that her school taught them in a residency to be humble as a doctor because it helps build your creditability. I wondered what she meant at first but then figured it out. What she was referring to is that a doctoral degree teaches you how to think first and to take in all the facts before you decide to say something. This is like the training you receive during your dissertation.

You learn to examine something closely before you speak to it. If you speak to it too soon because you assume that since you have the doctorate you could easily be lowering what your colleagues think of you and begin to lose creditability this way.

I've also learned quickly that there are a lot of people out there that have doctorates or PhD's that don't say anything or tell you unless you ask. I have a coworker that I recently found out has a PhD that I had no idea about. Modesty, humility, and humbleness can go a long way when dealing with other people if you don't try to push yourself on them because you have a doctorate or PhD. I have two other colleagues that are Dr's that prefer to not use their title unless it is strictly in a professional setting. I found this out when I referred to them as Dr. so and so and they politely asked me to call them by their first name. Both have had their degrees for some time and were kind enough to pass on their words of wisdom to me to help me along my path.

I only bring this topic up because this is a very big accomplishment for someone and it is nice to finish and walk across that stage, but many have gone before you and can teach you how to use constructively what you have achieved and not let you use it in a negative way. Believe me, I have seen people use it negatively in my past and I can see why my mentors pointed this out to me so that I don't make the same mistake.

My advice to you is to be careful after you "walk" because this is only the beginning of an adventure that has the potential to do big things for you and you don't want to spoil it. Don't let this accomplishment go to your head or you might find yourself behind the eight ball because of your thoughtlessness. Walk lightly with this accomplishment and the rest will fall into place for you as your career and life continue.

You can look at it like when you first got your driver's license. The day you got your license didn't make you the most experienced driver on the road but gave you the opportunity to really start learning about how to be a driver. It takes years before you become a good driver and learn things from experience. The same applies to getting your doctorate degree.

At one of my residencies, the facilitator told us that the dissertation is like your learner's permit, to learn how to conduct research. She told us that after you graduate it takes time to really absorb what you have learned and what you went through to get to that point. You don't become the expert right away because you just earned the title. Take your time and enhance the skills you have learned and really become a good doctor, not just a doctor.

Another way of looking at this is that you just made a very large investment in your future and the last thing you want to do with it is to not use it to your full advantage. A colleague once told me that they don't just give away doctorates or PhD's, you must go out and earn them and not everybody can do that. Anything worth working on is worth having so make sure that you take good care of your accomplishment.

So, the Doctoral Journey is just that, a journey into the unknown for a goal that is not easy to attain. A journey takes you on a path that is not charted, that has many unknowns but will take you to a destination that is worth getting to if you can make it through its uncharted ways.

There is nothing more rewarding than receiving acknowledgement that you have achieved a goal that you had to work hard for that will have an everlasting effect on your life as long as you are alive. The title "Doctor" becomes a permanent part of your life from the moment you receive it when you graduate and stays with you for the rest of your life.

I hope that this book helps in making the decision if pursuing a doctorate or PhD is the right thing for you. Many have entered this journey without the advantage of having a glimpse in to what the experience of the journey is about. This book is designed to give the perspective doctoral candidate just that glimpse. Good luck.

ABOUT THE AUTHOR

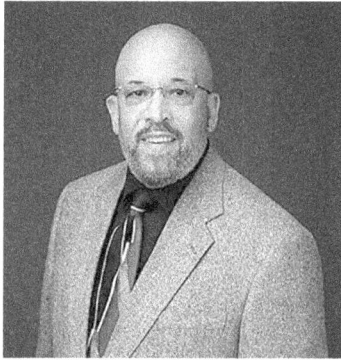

Dr. Evans was born and raised in Buffalo, N. Y. A 30-year Navy Veteran who retired in 2004, worked for the Navy after retirement as the Director of Public Health at Naval Hospital Camp Pendleton, California for 15 years. He completed his Doctoral Degree in Health Administration from The University of Phoenix in 2016 and holds several degrees in Healthcare and Business Management.

www.ingramcontent.com/pod-product-compliance
Lightning Source LLC
Chambersburg PA
CBHW032056040426
42335CB00036B/432